Yoga for Women's Reproductive Health

A No-Stress Exercise Plan with Easy Yoga Poses for a Healthy Uterus

Natural Solutions for Uterine Wellness, PCOS, and Menstrual Balance

BY

Sunita Jain

Table of Content

Introduction

Chapter 1: The Extreme Power of Yoga for Women's Reproductive Health

Introduction

For centuries, yoga has been revered for its transformative power to heal, balance, and harmonize the body, mind, and spirit. Today, women are discovering the profound benefits of yoga for their reproductive health. From alleviating menstrual cramps and bloating to enhancing fertility and hormonal balance, yoga offers a natural, holistic approach to wellness.

The Connection Between Yoga and Women's Reproductive Health

Yoga's impact on women's reproductive health stems from its ability to:

1. Balance Hormones: Yoga regulates hormone production, easing symptoms of PMS, PCOS, and menopause.

2. Strengthen the Pelvic Floor: Yoga tones the muscles supporting the uterus, bladder, and bowels.

3. Improve Blood Flow: Yoga enhances circulation to the reproductive organs, promoting healthy ovulation and menstruation.

4. Reduce Stress: Yoga calms the mind and body, mitigating stress's negative impact on reproductive health.

The Science Behind Yoga's Benefits

Research has shown that yoga:

1. Decreases cortisol levels, alleviating stress and anxiety.

2. Increases oxytocin, promoting & enhance feelings of relaxation and well-being.

3. Enhances insulin sensitivity, improving hormonal balance.

4. Supports immune function, reducing inflammation.

Key Principles for Practicing Yoga for Women's Reproductive Health

1. Listen to Your Body: Honor your unique needs and limitations.

2. Breathe and Relax: Cultivate calm and inner peace.

3. Move with Intention: Engage your core and pelvic floor.

4. Connect with Your Cycle: Attune your practice to your menstrual cycle.

Practice

Try this simple yoga sequence to connect with your body:

1. Mountain Pose (Tadasana)

2. Downward-Facing Dog (Adho Mukha Svanasana)

3. Cobra Pose (Bhujangasana)

4. Child's Pose (Balasana)

Conclusion

Yoga offers a powerful tool for transforming your reproductive health. By embracing this ancient practice, you'll unlock a deeper connection with your body, cultivate resilience, and radiate vibrant well-being.

Chapter 2: Understanding Women's Reproductive Health: Common Challenges and Concerns

Introduction

Women's reproductive health encompasses physical, emotional, and hormonal well-being. Understanding common challenges and concerns is crucial for empowered self-care.

Common Reproductive Health Challenges

1. Menstrual Irregularities: Infrequent, heavy, or painful periods.
2. Polycystic Ovary Syndrome (PCOS): Hormonal imbalance affecting ovulation and fertility.

3. Endometriosis: Painful condition where uterine tissue grows outside the uterus.

4. Fibroids: Benign tumors affecting uterine health.

5. Infertility: Difficulty conceiving.

6. Menopause: Hormonal changes during transition.

Hormonal Imbalance

1. Estrogen Dominance: Excess estrogen linked to mood swings, bloating, and weight gain.

2. Progesterone Deficiency: Low progesterone affecting ovulation and pregnancy.

3. Thyroid Hormone Imbalance: Impacting menstrual regularity and fertility.

Emotional and Psychological Concerns

1. Body Image Issues: Negative self-perception affecting self-esteem.

2. Anxiety and Depression: Mental health concerns impacting reproductive well-being.

3. Trauma and Stress: Adverse experiences affecting hormonal balance.

Factors Influencing Reproductive Health

1. Genetics: Family history and genetic predispositions.
2. Lifestyle Choices: Diet, exercise, and stress management.
3. Environmental Toxins: Exposure to endocrine-disrupting chemicals.
4. Age: Reproductive health changes across lifespan.

Breaking the Silence

Sharing personal experiences and concerns with healthcare providers, loved ones, or support groups can:

1. Reduce stigma
2. Increase awareness
3. Foster empathy
4. Encourage empowerment

Practice

Try this simple breathing exercise to calm your mind and body into a proper relaxation:

1. Deep inhale through nose (4 counts)
2. Hold breath (4 counts)
3. Slow exhale through mouth (4 counts)
4. Repeat (3-5 cycles)

Conclusion

Understanding common reproductive health challenges and concerns is the first step toward empowerment. By acknowledging these issues, you'll better navigate your own reproductive journey.

Part 1: Foundations of Yoga for Women's Reproductive Health

Chapter 3: Yoga Philosophy and Women's Health: A Holistic Approach

Introduction

Yoga's ancient philosophy offers a profound framework for understanding women's health. By integrating physical, mental, and spiritual practices, yoga fosters holistic well-being.

Key Yoga Philosophies for Women's Health

1. Ahimsa (Non-Violence): Self-care and compassion.
2. Pratihara (Withdrawal of the Senses): Mindfulness and introspection.
3. Prana (Life Force): Balancing energy for vitality.
4. Dinacharya (Daily Routine): Harmonizing daily rhythms.

The Five Koshas (Sheaths) and Women's Health

1. Annamaya Kosha (Physical Body): Nourishment and movement.

2. Pranamaya Kosha (Energetic Body): Breath and vitality.

3. Manomaya Kosha (Mental Body): Emotional balance and clarity.

4. Vijnanamaya Kosha (Intuitive Body): Inner wisdom and guidance.

5. Anandamaya Kosha (Blissful Body): Connection to inner joy.

Yoga's Holistic Approach to Women's Health

1. Physical Postures (Asanas): Strengthening and balancing.

2. Breath Awareness (Pranayama): Regulating hormones and emotions.

3. Meditation and Relaxation: Calming the mind and body.

4. Lifestyle and Rituals: Nourishing body, mind, and spirit.

The Three Gunas and Women's Health

1. Sattva (Balance): Harmony and equilibrium.
2. Rajas (Activity): Energy and dynamism.
3. Tamas (Inertia): Rest and rejuvenation.

Applying Yoga Philosophy to Women's Health Concerns

1. Menstrual health: Harnessing prana and balancing hormones.
2. Fertility: Cultivating sattva and inner balance.
3. Menopause: Embracing transformation and inner wisdom.

Practice

Try this simple yoga sequence to cultivate balance:

1. Mountain Pose (Tadasana)
2. Downward-Facing Dog (Adho Mukha Svanasana)
3. Warrior Pose (Virabhadrasana)
4. Seated Forward Fold (Paschimottanasana)

Conclusion

Yoga philosophy provides a profound framework for understanding women's health. By embracing this holistic approach, you'll cultivate balance, vitality, and inner harmony.

Chapter 4: Breathing Techniques for Hormonal Balance and Relaxation

Introduction

Breath is life. Conscious breathing techniques can harmonize hormones, calm the mind, and soothe the body. Discover how to harness the power of breath for optimal well-being.

The Science of Breath and Hormones

1. Stress and Cortisol: How breathing affects hormone regulation.

2. Oxytocin and Relaxation: Breath's role in releasing "feel-good" hormones.

3. Endocrine System and Breath: Balancing hormones through respiratory rhythms.

Breathing Techniques for Hormonal Balance

1. Diaphragmatic Breathing: Engaging the lower lungs for relaxation.

2. Alternate Nostril Breathing: Balancing left and right brain hemispheres.

3. Kapalabhati Breathing: Stimulating digestive and endocrine systems.

4. Bhastrika Breathing: Energizing and balancing hormones.

Breathing Techniques for Relaxation and Stress Relief

1. 4-7-8 Breathing: Calming the nervous system.

2. Box Breathing: Focusing the mind and calming emotions.

3. Progressive Muscle Relaxation: Releasing physical tension.

4. Visualization and Breath: Guided imagery for relaxation.

Women-Specific Breathing Techniques

1. Menstrual Cycle Breathing: Harmonizing breath with menstrual rhythms.
2. Fertility Breathing: Enhancing reproductive health.
3. Menopause Breathing: Managing symptoms and stress.

Tips for Effective Breathing Practice

1. Start small: Begin with short sessions.
2. Consistency; Practice daily.
3. Focus: Concentrate on breath.
4. Relaxation: Release tension.

Real-Life Examples and Success Stories

Meet Sally, who reduced stress and balanced hormones with breathing techniques:

"Breathing changed my life. I feel more centered and calm."

Practice

Try this simple breathing exercise:

1. Inhale deeply through nose (4 counts)

2. Hold breath (4 counts)

3. Exhale slowly through mouth (4 counts)

4. Repeat (3-5 cycles)

Conclusion

Conscious breathing transforms lives. By harnessing the power of breath, you'll balance hormones, relax, and radiate vibrant well-being.

Chapter 5: Foundational Yoga Poses for Women's Reproductive Health

Introduction

Yoga postures (asanas) can profoundly impact women's reproductive health. This chapter explores foundational poses to cultivate balance, strength, and flexibility.

Benefits of Yoga for Women's Reproductive Health

1. Hormonal Balance: Yoga regulates hormone production.

2. Pelvic Floor Strength: Yoga tones muscles supporting the uterus.

3. Menstrual Health: Yoga eases cramps, bloating, and mood swings.

4. Fertility: Yoga enhances reproductive function.

Foundational Yoga Poses for Women's Reproductive Health

Section 1: Pelvic Floor Strengthening

1. Mountain Pose (Tadasana): Establishes core strength.

2. Downward-Facing Dog (Adho Mukha Svanasana): Stretches and strengthens pelvic floor.

3. Squats (Malasana): Tones uterus-supporting muscles.

Section 2: Hormonal Balance and Relaxation

1. Child's Pose (Balasana): Calms nervous system.

2. Seated Forward Fold (Paschimottanasana): Stretches endocrine system.

3. Legs Up The Wall Pose (Viparita Karani): Inverts uterus, promoting relaxation.

Section 3: Menstrual Health and Cramp Relief

1. Cobra Pose (Bhujangasana): Opens chest, easing respiratory tension.

2. Cat-Cow Pose (Marjaryasana-Bitilasana): Warms spinal fluid, reducing cramps.

3. Reclined Pigeon Pose (Supta Eka Pada Rajakapotasana): Relaxes lower back.

Section 4: Fertility and Reproductive Health

1. Butterfly Pose (Baddha Konasana): Stimulates ovaries.

2. Seated Twist (Bharadvajasana): Enhances spinal flexibility.

3. Savasana (Corpse Pose): Cultivates relaxation, essential for fertility.

Tips for Practicing Yoga during Menstruation

1. Listen to your body: Modify or rest when needed.

2. Avoid inverted poses: Unless specifically recommended.

3. Prioritize relaxation: Focus on calming postures.

Real-Life Examples and Success Stories

Meet Andrea, who alleviated menstrual cramps with yoga:

"Yoga transformed my periods. I feel empowered and pain-free."

Practice

Try this simple yoga sequence:

1. Mountain Pose (Tadasana)
2. Downward-Facing Dog (Adho Mukha Svanasana)
3. Child's Pose (Balasana)
4. Seated Forward Fold (Paschimottanasana)

Conclusion

Foundational yoga poses lay the groundwork for optimal women's reproductive health. By practicing these postures, you'll cultivate balance, strength, and flexibility.

Part 2: Yoga for Uterine Wellness

Chapter 6: Yoga for Uterine Health: Strengthening the Core and Pelvic Floor

Introduction

A healthy uterus relies on a strong core and pelvic floor. Yoga offers targeted practices to tone these muscles, enhancing uterine well-being.

The Importance & prominence of Core and Pelvic Floor Strength

1. Uterine Support: Strong muscles reduce prolapse risk.

2. Menstrual Health: Strengthened pelvic floor eases cramps and heavy bleeding.

3. Fertility: Optimal uterine positioning enhances reproductive function.

4. Bladder Control: Pelvic floor strength prevents incontinence.

Yoga Poses for Core Strength

1. Plank Pose (Phalakasana): Engages entire core.

2. Boat Pose (Paripurna Navasana): Strengthens abdominal muscles.

3. Side Plank Pose (Vasisthasana): Targets obliques.

Yoga Poses for Pelvic Floor Strength

1. Mula Bandha: Engages pelvic floor muscles.

2. Squats (Malasana): Tones uterus-supporting muscles.

3. Bridge Pose (Setu Bandha Sarvangasana): Strengthens pelvic floor.

Yoga Sequences for Uterine Health

Sequence 1: Uterine Support

1. Mountain Pose (Tadasana)

2. Downward-Facing Dog (Adho Mukha Svanasana)

3. Plank Pose (Phalakasana)

4. Squats (Malasana)

Sequence 2: Menstrual Health

1. Child's Pose (Balasana)

2. Seated Forward Fold (Paschimottanasana)

3. Reclined (Lean Back)Pigeon Pose (Supta Eka Pada Rajakapotasana)

4. Legs Up(Bunk-up) The Wall Pose (Viparita Karani)

Tips for Practicing Yoga during Uterine Health Concerns

1. Listen to your body: Modify or rest when needed.

2. Avoid deep twists: Unless specifically recommended.

3. Prioritize relaxation: Focus on calming postures.

Real-Life Examples and Success Stories

Meet Sandy, who strengthened her pelvic floor with yoga:

"Yoga transformed my uterine health. I feel empowered and confident."

Practice

Try this simple yoga sequence:

1. Mountain Pose (Tadasana)
2. Downward-Facing Dog (Adho Mukha Svanasana)
3. Plank Pose (Phalakasana)
4. Squats (Malasana)

Conclusion

Yoga offers a powerful tool for enhancing uterine health. By strengthening your core and pelvic floor, you'll cultivate optimal well-being.

Chapter 7: Yoga for Menstrual Balance: Regulating the Cycle

Introduction

Menstrual balance is essential for women's health. Yoga offers targeted practices to regulate the cycle, alleviate symptoms, and enhance overall well-being.

The Benefits of Yoga for Menstrual Balance

1. Regulates Hormones: Yoga balances estrogen and progesterone.

2. Eases Cramps: Yoga reduces menstrual pain.

3. Improves Mood: Yoga alleviates anxiety and depression.

4. Enhances Fertility: Yoga optimizes reproductive health.

Yoga Poses for Menstrual Balance

Section 1: Hormone Regulation

1. Downward-Facing Dog (Adho Mukha Svanasana): Balances endocrine system.

2. Seated Forward Fold (Paschimottanasana): Stimulates hormone production.

3. Plow Pose (Halasana): Regulates thyroid function.

Section 2: Cramp Relief

1. Child's Pose (Balasana): Soothes lower back.

2. Reclined Pigeon Pose (Supta Eka Pada Rajakapotasana): Relaxes pelvic muscles.

3. Sphinx Pose (Salamba Bhujangasana): Opens chest, easing respiratory tension.

Section 3: Mood Enhancement

1. Sun Salutations (Surya Namaskar): Boosts mood and energy.

2. Legs Up The Wall Pose (Viparita Karani): Calms nervous system.

3. Savasana (Corpse Pose): Reduces stress and anxiety.

Yoga Sequences for Menstrual Balance

Sequence 1: Menstrual Regulation

1. Downward-Facing Dog (Adho Mukha Svanasana)
2. Seated Forward Fold (Paschimottanasana)
3. Plow Pose (Halasana)
4. Child's Pose (Balasana)

Sequence 2: Cramp Relief

1. Reclined Pigeon Pose (Supta Eka Pada Rajakapotasana)
2. Sphinx Pose (Salamba Bhujangasana)
3. Seated Twist (Bharadvajasana)
4. Savasana (Corpse Pose)

Tips for Practising Yoga during Menstruation

1. Listen to your body: Modify or rest when needed.

2. Avoid inverted poses: Unless specifically recommended.

3. Prioritise relaxation: Focus on calming postures.

Real-Life Examples and Success Stories

Meet Abby, who regulated her cycle with yoga:

"Yoga transformed my periods. I feel balanced and empowered."

Practice

Try this simple yoga sequence:

1. Downward-Facing Dog (Adho Mukha Svanasana)

2. Seated Forward Fold (Paschimottanasana)

3. Child's Pose (Balasana)

4. Savasana (Corpse Pose)

Conclusion

Yoga offers a natural solution for menstrual balance. By incorporating these practices, you'll regulate your cycle, alleviate symptoms, and enhance overall well-being.

Chapter 8: Yoga for Fibroids and Endometriosis: Relief and Management

Introduction

Fibroids and endometriosis affect millions of women worldwide. Yoga offers a holistic approach to managing symptoms, reducing pain, and enhancing overall well-being.

Understanding Fibroids and Endometriosis

1. Fibroids: Benign tumors growing in the uterus.
2. Endometriosis: Uterine tissue growing outside the uterus.

Yoga Benefits for Fibroids and Endometriosis

1. Reduces Pain: Yoga alleviates cramping and discomfort.

2. Regulates Hormones: Yoga balances oestrogen and progesterone.

3. Improves Circulation: Yoga enhances blood flow to the pelvis.

4. Reduces Stress: Yoga calms the mind and body.

Yoga Poses for Fibroid Relief

1. Child's Pose (Balasana): Soothes lower back.

2. Reclined Pigeon Pose (Supta Eka Pada Rajakapotasana): Relaxes pelvic muscles.

3. Sphinx Pose (Salamba Bhujangasana): Opens chest, easing respiratory tension.

4. Legs Up The Wall Pose (Viparita Karani): Inverts uterus, reducing pressure.

Yoga Poses for Endometriosis Relief

1. Downward-Facing Dog (Adho Mukha Svanasana): Balances endocrine system.

2. Seated Forward Fold (Paschimottanasana): Stimulates hormone production.

3. Plow Pose (Halasana): Regulates thyroid function.

4. Savasana (Corpse Pose): Reduces stress and anxiety.

Yoga Sequences for Fibroid and Endometriosis Management

Sequence 1: Fibroid Relief

1. Child's Pose (Balasana)
2. Reclined Pigeon Pose (Supta Eka Pada Rajakapotasana)
3. Sphinx Pose (Salamba Bhujangasana)
4. Legs Up (Bunk-up) The Wall Pose (Viparita Karani)

Sequence 2: Endometriosis Relief

1. Downward-Facing Dog (Adho Mukha Svanasana)
2. Seated Forward Fold (Paschimottanasana)
3. Plow Pose (Halasana)
4. Savasana (Corpse Pose)

Breathing Techniques and Relaxation

1. Alternate Nostril Breathing: Balances left and right brain hemispheres.

2. Progressive Muscle Relaxation: Releases physical tension.

3. Visualization: Guided imagery for relaxation.

Real-Life Examples and Success Stories

Meet Tilly, who managed fibroid symptoms with yoga:

"Yoga extremely reduced my pain and improved my overall well-being."

Practice

Try this simple yoga sequence:

1. Child's Pose (Balasana)

2. Downward-Facing Dog (Adho Mukha Svanasana)

3. Seated Forward Fold (Paschimottanasana)

4. Savasana (Corpse Pose)

Conclusion

Yoga offers a holistic approach to managing fibroids and endometriosis. By incorporating these practices, you'll reduce symptoms, enhance overall well-being, and cultivate resilience.

Part 3: Yoga for PCOS and Hormonal Balance

Chapter 9: Understanding PCOS: Causes, Symptoms, and Yoga Solutions

Introduction

Polycystic Ovary Syndrome (PCOS) affects millions & millions of women worldwide. Yoga offers a holistic approach to managing symptoms, balancing hormones, and enhancing overall well-being.

Understanding PCOS

1. Definition: Hormonal disorder affecting ovulation and fertility.
2. Causes: Genetic, environmental, and lifestyle factors.
3. Symptoms: Irregular periods, weight gain, acne, and infertility.

Common PCOS Symptoms

1. Hormonal Imbalance: Androgen excess, insulin resistance.

2. Menstrual Irregularities: Infrequent or absent periods.

3. Weight Management: Difficulty losing weight.

4. Skin Issues: Acne, hair loss.

Yoga Benefits for PCOS

1. Hormone Regulation: Yoga balances cortisol, insulin, and androgen.

2. Weight Management: Yoga enhances metabolism, reduces stress.

3. Menstrual Regularity: Yoga regulates ovulation, improves fertility.

4. Stress Reduction: Yoga calms mind and body.

Yoga Poses for PCOS

1. Downward-Facing Dog (Adho Mukha Svanasana): Balances endocrine system.

2. Warrior Pose (Virabhadrasana): Enhances insulin sensitivity.

3. Triangle Pose (Trikonasana): Stimulates ovarian function.

4. Seated Forward Fold (Paschimottanasana): Regulates menstrual cycle.

Yoga Sequences for PCOS Management

Sequence 1: Hormone Balance

1. Downward-Facing Dog (Adho Mukha Svanasana)

2. Warrior Pose (Virabhadrasana)

3. Triangle Pose (Trikonasana)

4. Seated Forward Fold (Paschimottanasana)

Sequence 2: Weight Management

1. Sun Salutations (Surya Namaskar)

2. Plank Pose (Phalakasana)

3. Boat Pose (Paripurna Navasana)

4. Legs Up(Bunk-up) The Wall Pose (Viparita Karani)

Breathing Techniques and Relaxation

1. Alternate Nostril Breathing: Balances left and right brain hemispheres.

2. Progressive Muscle Relaxation: Releases physical tension.

3. Visualisation: Guided imagery for relaxation.

Practice

Try this simple yoga sequence:

1. Downward-Facing Dog (Adho Mukha Svanasana)

2. Warrior Pose (Virabhadrasana)

3. Seated Forward Fold (Paschimottanasana)

4. Savasana (Corpse Pose)

Conclusion

Yoga offers a holistic approach to managing PCOS. By incorporating these practices, you'll balance hormones, regulate menstrual cycles, and enhance overall well-being.

Chapter 10: Yoga for Hormonal Balance: Regulating Insulin and Testosterone

Introduction

Hormonal balance is crucial for overall health. Yoga offers targeted practices to regulate insulin and testosterone, alleviating symptoms associated with hormonal imbalances.

Understanding Insulin Resistance and Testosterone Imbalance

1. Insulin Resistance: Precursor to diabetes and metabolic syndrome.
2. Testosterone Imbalance: Affects fertility, energy, and mood.

Yoga Benefits for Hormonal Balance

1. Regulates Blood Sugar: Yoga enhances insulin sensitivity.

2. Balances Testosterone: Yoga reduces symptoms of excess testosterone.

3. Reduces Stress: Yoga calms mind and body.

Yoga Poses for Insulin Regulation

1. Downward-Facing Dog (Adho Mukha Svanasana): Enhances insulin sensitivity.

2. Warrior Pose (Virabhadrasana): Stimulates glucose uptake.

3. Triangle Pose (Trikonasana): Balances pancreatic function.

4. Seated Forward Fold (Paschimottanasana): Regulates blood sugar.

Yoga Poses for Testosterone Balance

1. Plank Pose (Phalakasana): Strengthens adrenal glands.

2. Cobra Pose (Bhujangasana): Stimulates testosterone production.

3. Seated Twist (Bharadvajasana): Balances hormone regulation.

4. Savasana (Corpse Pose): Reduces stress and cortisol.

Yoga Sequences for Hormonal Balance

Sequence 1: Insulin Regulation

1. Downward-Facing Dog (Adho Mukha Svanasana)

2. Warrior Pose (Virabhadrasana)

3. Triangle Pose (Trikonasana)

4. Seated Forward Fold (Paschimottanasana)

Sequence 2: Testosterone Balance

1. Plank Pose (Phalakasana)

2. Cobra Pose (Bhujangasana)

3. Seated Twist (Bharadvajasana)

4. Savasana (Corpse Pose)

Breathing Techniques and Relaxation

1. Alternate Nostril Breathing: Balances left and right brain hemispheres.
2. Progressive Muscle Relaxation: Releases physical tension.
3. Visualisation: Guided imagery for relaxation.

Practice

Try this simple yoga sequence:

1. Downward-Facing Dog (Adho Mukha Svanasana)
2. Warrior Pose (Virabhadrasana)
3. Seated Forward Fold (Paschimottanasana)
4. Savasana (Corpse Pose)

Conclusion

Yoga offers a holistic (systemic) approach to regulating & control insulin and testosterone. By incorporating these practices, you'll balance hormones, alleviate symptoms, and enhance overall well-being.

Chapter 11: Yoga for Weight Management and PCOS

Introduction

Weight management is crucial for overall health, especially for women with Polycystic Ovary Syndrome (PCOS). Yoga offers targeted practices to regulate weight, balance hormones, and alleviate PCOS symptoms.

Understanding Weight Management and PCOS

1. PCOS and Weight Gain: Hormonal imbalance and insulin resistance.
2. Weight Loss Challenges: Metabolic slowdown and emotional eating.

Yoga Benefits for Weight Management and PCOS

1. Regulates Metabolism: Yoga enhances insulin sensitivity.

2. Balances Hormones: Yoga reduces androgen excess.

3. Reduces Stress: Yoga calms mind and body.

4. Improves Body Image: Yoga promotes self-acceptance.

Yoga Poses for Weight Management

1. Sun Salutations (Surya Namaskar): Boosts metabolism.

2. Warrior Pose (Virabhadrasana): Strengthens muscles.

3. Triangle Pose (Trikonasana): Stimulates digestion.

4. Downward-Facing Dog (Adho Mukha Svanasana): Enhances insulin sensitivity.

Yoga Poses for PCOS Weight Management

1. Plank Pose (Phalakasana): Strengthens core and balances hormones.

2. Seated Forward Fold (Paschimottanasana): Regulates menstrual cycle.

3. Seated Twist (Bharadvajasana): Balances hormone regulation.

4. Savasana (Corpse Pose): Reduces stress and cortisol.

Yoga Sequences for Weight Management and PCOS

Sequence 1: Weight Loss

1. Sun Salutations (Surya Namaskar)

2. Warrior Pose (Virabhadrasana)

3. Triangle Pose (Trikonasana)

4. Downward-Facing Dog (Adho Mukha Svanasana)

Sequence 2: PCOS Weight Management

1. Plank Pose (Phalakasana)

2. Seated Forward Fold (Paschimottanasana)

3. Seated Twist (Bharadvajasana)

4. Savasana (Corpse Pose)

Breathing Techniques and Relaxation

1. Alternate Nostril Breathing: Balances left and right brain hemispheres.

2. Progressive Muscle Relaxation: Releases physical tension.

3. Visualisation: Guided imagery for relaxation.

Practice

Try this simple yoga sequence:

1. Sun Salutations (Surya Namaskar)

2. Warrior Pose (Virabhadrasana)

3. Seated Forward Fold (Paschimottanasana)

4. Savasana (Corpse Pose)

Conclusion

Yoga offers a holistic approach to weight management and PCOS. By incorporating these practices, you'll regulate weight, balance hormones, and alleviate symptoms.

Part 4: Yoga for Menstrual Wellness

Chapter 12: Yoga for Menstrual Cramps and PMS Relief

Introduction

Menstrual cramps and Premenstrual Syndrome (PMS) affect millions of women worldwide. Yoga offers targeted practices to alleviate symptoms, reduce pain, and enhance overall well-being.

Understanding Menstrual Cramps and PMS

1. Menstrual Cramps: Uterine contractions causing pain.
2. PMS: Hormonal changes leading to physical and emotional symptoms.

Yoga Benefits for Menstrual Cramps and PMS Relief

1. Reduces Pain: Yoga relaxes uterine muscles.

2. Regulates Hormones: Yoga balances oestrogen and progesterone.

3. Eases Symptoms: Yoga alleviates bloating, mood swings.

4. Enhances Well-being: Yoga promotes relaxation and self-awareness.

Yoga Poses for Menstrual Cramp Relief

1. Child's Pose (Balasana): Soothes lower back.

2. Reclined Pigeon Pose (Supta Eka Pada Rajakapotasana): Relaxes pelvic muscles.

3. Sphinx Pose (Salamba Bhujangasana): Opens chest, easing respiratory tension.

4. Legs Up The Wall Pose (Viparita Karani): Inverts uterus, reducing pressure.

Yoga Poses for PMS Relief

1. (Dog-like pose) Downward-Facing Dog (Adho Mukha Svanasana): Balances endocrine system.

2. Seated Forward Fold (Paschimottanasana): Stimulates hormone production.

3. Plow Pose (Halasana): Regulates thyroid function.

4. Savasana (Corpse Pose): Reduces stress and anxiety.

Yoga Sequences for Menstrual Cramp and PMS Relief

Sequence 1: Menstrual Cramp Relief

1. Child's Pose (Balasana)
2. Reclined(Lean Back) Pigeon Pose (Supta Eka Pada Rajakapotasana)
3. Sphinx Pose (Salamba Bhujangasana)
4. Legs Up(Bunk-up) The Wall Pose (Viparita Karani)

Sequence 2: PMS Relief

1. Downward-Facing Dog (Adho Mukha Svanasana)
2. Seated Forward Fold (Paschimottanasana)
3. Plow Pose (Halasana)
4. Savasana (Corpse Pose)

Breathing Techniques and Relaxation

1. Alternate Nostril Breathing: Balances left and right brain hemispheres.

2. Progressive Muscle Relaxation: Releases physical tension.

3. Visualisation: Guided imagery for relaxation.

Practice

Try this simple yoga sequence:

1. Child's Pose (Balasana)

2. Downward-Facing Dog (Adho Mukha Svanasana)

3. Seated Forward Fold (Paschimottanasana)

4. Savasana (Corpse Pose)

Conclusion

Yoga offers a natural solution for menstrual cramp and PMS relief. By incorporating these practices, you'll reduce symptoms, enhance well-being, and cultivate resilience.

Chapter 13: Yoga for Menstrual Irregularities: Regulating the Cycle

Introduction

Menstrual irregularities affect millions of women worldwide. Yoga offers targeted practices to regulate the cycle, balance hormones, and enhance reproductive health.

Understanding Menstrual Irregularities

1. Amenorrhea: Absence of menstruation.

2. Oligomenorrhea: Infrequent menstruation.

3. Polymenorrhea: Frequent menstruation.

4. Dysmenorrhea: Painful menstruation.

Yoga Benefits for Menstrual Regularity

1. Regulates Hormones: Yoga balances oestrogen and progesterone.

2. Enhances Fertility: Yoga optimises reproductive health.

3. Reduces Stress: Yoga calms mind and body.

4. Improves Menstrual Cycle: Yoga regulates ovulation and menstruation.

Yoga Poses for Menstrual Regularity

1. Downward-Facing Dog (Adho Mukha Svanasana): Balances endocrine system.

2. Seated Forward Fold (Paschimottanasana): Stimulates hormone production.

3. Plow Pose (Halasana): Regulates thyroid function.

4. Sphinx Pose (Salamba Bhujangasana): Enhances ovarian function.

Yoga Sequences for Menstrual Regularity

Sequence 1: Hormone Balance

1. Downward-Facing Dog (Adho Mukha Svanasana)
2. Seated Forward Fold (Paschimottanasana)
3. Plow Pose (Halasana)
4. Sphinx Pose (Salamba Bhujangasana)

Sequence 2: Menstrual Regulation

1. Child's Pose (Balasana)
2. Reclined(Lean back) Pigeon Pose (Supta Eka Pada Rajakapotasana)
3. Seated Twist (Bharadvajasana)
4. Savasana (Corpse Pose)

Breathing Techniques and Relaxation

1. Alternate Nostril Breathing: Balances left and right brain hemispheres.
2. Progressive Muscle Relaxation: Releases physical tension.
3. Visualisation: Guided imagery for relaxation.

Practice

Try this simple yoga sequence:

1. Downward-Facing Dog (Adho Mukha Svanasana)
2. Seated Forward Fold (Paschimottanasana)
3. Sphinx Pose (Salamba Bhujangasana)
4. Savasana (Corpse Pose)

Conclusion

Yoga offers a holistic approach to regulating menstrual irregularities. By incorporating these practices, you'll balance hormones, enhance reproductive health, and cultivate overall well-being.

Chapter 14: Yoga for Perimenopause and Menopause Transition

Introduction

Perimenopause and menopause mark significant changes in a woman's life. Yoga offers targeted practices to alleviate symptoms, balance hormones, and enhance overall well-being.

Understanding Perimenopause and Menopause

1. Perimenopause: Transitional phase before menopause.

2. Menopause: Cessation of menstruation.

3. Symptoms: Hot flashes, night sweats, mood swings.

Yoga Benefits for Perimenopause and Menopause

1. Reduces Symptoms: Yoga alleviates hot flashes, night sweats.

2. Balances Hormones: Yoga regulates oestrogen and progesterone.

3. Enhances Bone Density: Yoga reduces osteoporosis risk.

4. Improves Mental Health: Yoga reduces anxiety, depression.

Yoga Poses for Perimenopause and Menopause

1. Downward-Facing Dog (Adho Mukha Svanasana): Balances endocrine system.

2. Seated Forward Fold (Paschimottanasana): Stimulates hormone production.

3. Warrior Pose (Virabhadrasana): Strengthens bones.

4. Savasana (Corpse Pose): Reduces stress and anxiety.

Yoga Sequences for Perimenopause and Menopause

Sequence 1: Hormone Balance

1. Downward-Facing Dog (Adho Mukha Svanasana)
2. Seated Forward Fold (Paschimottanasana)
3. Plow Pose (Halasana)
4. Sphinx Pose (Salamba Bhujangasana)

Sequence 2: Symptom Relief

1. Child's Pose (Balasana)
2. Reclined(Lean Back) Pigeon Pose (Supta Eka Pada Rajakapotasana)
3. Seated Twist (Bharadvajasana)
4. Legs Up(Bunk-up) The Wall Pose (Viparita Karani)

Breathing Techniques and Relaxation

1. Alternate Nostril Breathing: Balances left and right brain hemispheres.
2. Progressive Muscle Relaxation: Releases physical tension.
3. Visualisation: Guided imagery for relaxation.

Practice

Try this simple yoga sequence:

1. Downward-Facing Dog (Adho Mukha Svanasana)
2. Seated Forward Fold (Paschimottanasana)
3. Warrior Pose (Virabhadrasana)
4. Savasana (Corpse Pose)

Conclusion

Yoga offers a (systemic) holistic approach to navigating perimenopause and menopause. By incorporating these practices, you'll balance hormones, alleviate symptoms, and cultivate overall well-being.

Part 5: Advanced Yoga Practices and Lifestyle Changes

Chapter 15: Advanced Yoga Techniques for Women's Reproductive Health(Uterus)

Introduction

Building on the foundational practices, this chapter explores advanced yoga techniques to optimise women's reproductive health.

Advanced Yoga Techniques

1. Bandha (Energy Locks): Engage Mula Bandha (root lock) to stimulate pelvic floor muscles.
2. Mudras (Hand Gestures): Practise Prana Mudra to balance life force energy.
3. Pranayama (Breath Control): Use Bhastrika (bellows breath) to stimulate hormone production.

4. Kundalini Yoga: Activate energy through postures, breath, and meditation.

Yoga for Specific Reproductive Concerns

1. Endometriosis: Focus on pelvic floor strengthening and hormone regulation.
2. Fibroids: Practise uterine-toning postures and breathwork.
3. PCOS: Balance insulin and hormone regulation through targeted practices.
4. Menopause: Use yoga to alleviate symptoms and enhance bone density.

Advanced Sequences

Sequence 1: Hormone Balance

1. Downward-Facing Dog (Adho Mukha Svanasana)
2. Seated Forward Fold (Paschimottanasana)
3. Plow Pose (Halasana)
4. Sphinx Pose (Salamba Bhujangasana)

Sequence 2: Reproductive Health

1. Cobra Pose (Bhujangasana)

2. Bow Pose (Dhanurasana)

3. Seated Twist (Bharadvajasana)

4. Savasana (Corpse Pose)

Meditation and Visualization

1. Guided imagery for reproductive health

2. Visualisation for hormone balance

3. Kundalini meditation for energy activation

Practice

Try this advanced yoga sequence:

1. Downward-Facing Dog (Adho Mukha Svanasana)

2. Cobra Pose (Bhujangasana)

3. Seated Forward Fold (Paschimottanasana)

4. Kundalini meditation

Conclusion

Advanced yoga techniques offer a powerful tool for optimising women's reproductive health. By incorporating these practices, you'll enhance hormone balance, alleviate symptoms, and cultivate overall well-being.

Chapter 16: Nutrition and Lifestyle Changes for Optimal Reproductive Health

Introduction

A balanced diet and healthy lifestyle are crucial for optimal reproductive health. This chapter explores nutrition and lifestyle changes to support hormone balance, fertility, and overall well-being.

Nutrition for Reproductive Health

1. Whole(unprocessed) Foods: Focus on organic fruits, vegetables, whole grains.
2. Omega-3 Rich Foods: Support hormone production with fatty fish, flaxseeds.
3. Antioxidant-Rich Foods: Berries, leafy greens reduce oxidative stress.

4. Probiotic-Rich Foods: Support gut health with yogurt, kefir, kimchi.

Foods to Avoid

1. Processed Foods: Limit sugary, packaged foods.

2. Soy and Phytoestrogens: May disrupt hormone balance.

3. Caffeine and Alcohol: Limit or avoid optimal fertility.

Lifestyle Changes for Reproductive Health

1. Stress Management: Yoga, meditation, deep breathing.

2. Exercise: Balance physical activity with rest and relaxation.

3. Sleep: Prioritise 7-8 hours of sleep per night.

4. Environmental Toxins: Avoid endocrine-disrupting chemicals.

Specific Dietary Recommendations

1. PCOS: Focus on insulin-sensitising foods, omega-3s.

2. Endometriosis: Increase antioxidant intake, reduce inflammation.

3. Menopause: Support bone health with calcium, vitamin D.

Lifestyle Tips for Specific Concerns

1. Fertility: Maintain healthy weight, manage stress.

2. Menstrual Health: Practise self-care during menstruation.

3. Pregnancy: Focus on prenatal nutrition, safe exercise.

Practice

Try these simple changes:

1. Incorporate omega-3 rich foods into your diet.

2. Practise deep breathing exercises daily.

3. Prioritise 7-8 hours of sleep per night.

Conclusion

Nutrition and lifestyle changes play a critical role in optimal reproductive health. By incorporating these changes, you'll enhance hormone balance, fertility, and overall well-being.

Chapter 17: How to have a healthy strong uterus speedily

Introduction

Mindfulness and stress management are essential for women's overall wellbeing. This chapter explores practical techniques to reduce stress, cultivate self-awareness, and enhance emotional resilience.

Benefits of Mindfulness for Women

1. Reduces stress and anxiety
2. Enhances emotional regulation
3. Improves self-awareness and self-acceptance
4. Supports physical health and wellbeing

Mindfulness Techniques for Women

1. Meditation: Focus on breath, body, or emotions

2. Deep Breathing: Calm nervous system and reduce stress

3. Yoga: Combine physical movement with mindfulness

Stress Management Strategies for Women

1. Prioritise Self-Care: Make(a good schedule)time for relaxation and pleasure

2. Set (limits) Clear Clean Boundaries: Learn to say "no" and maintain healthy relationships by setting limits.

3. Strongly Exercise often: Regular physical activity reduces stress and anxiety

4. Connect(Link) with Nature: Spend time outdoors to calm mind and body

Emotional Resilience Techniques

1. Grounding Techniques: Focus on present moment

2. Self-Compassion: Practice kindness and understanding towards oneself

Practice

Try these simple mindfulness exercises:

1. 5-minute meditation session daily
2. Deep breathing exercises before bed
3. Mindful walking or yoga practice

Conclusion

Mindfulness and stress management are powerful tools for women's wellbeing. By incorporating these techniques, you'll cultivate emotional resilience, reduce stress, and enhance overall wellbeing.

Conclusion

Healthy Uterus

Chapter 18: Integrating Yoga Uterus into Your Life: A Path to Long-Term Wellness

Introduction

Yoga is a journey, not a destination. This chapter explores practical ways to integrate yoga into daily life, ensuring long-term wellness and self-transformation.

Creating a Home Yoga Practice

1. Designate a perfect yoga space: Quiet, peaceful, and clutter-free
2. Set a regular schedule: Start small, aim for consistency
3. Begin with simple routines: Follow online classes or DVDs

4. Experiment with different styles: Find what resonates with you

Incorporating Yoga into Daily Activities

1. Morning yoga routine: Boost energy and clarity
2. Desk yoga: Reduce stress, improve focus
3. Yoga for travel: Stay flexible, relaxed on-the-go
4. Yoga for daily tasks: Mindful movement in everyday activities

Yoga Philosophy in Daily Life

1. Ahimsa (Non-Violence): Practise self-compassion, kindness
2. Satya (Truthfulness): Cultivate honesty, authenticity
3. Svadhyaya (Self-Study): Reflect, journal, and grow
4. Ishvara Pranidhana (Surrender): Let go, trust the process

Overcoming Obstacles and Staying Motivated

1. Find community support: Join yoga classes, workshops

2. Set realistic goals: Progress, not perfection

3. Mix it up: Try new styles, teachers, and practices

4. Self-care: Prioritise rest, relaxation, and rejuvenation

Practice

Try these simple integrations:

1. 5-minute morning yoga routine

2. Desk yoga breaks throughout the day

3. Mindful walking or eating

Conclusion

By integrating yoga into daily life, you'll cultivate long-term wellness, resilience, and radiant living.

Chapter 19: Conclusion: Empowering Women's Reproductive Health through Yoga

Introduction

As we conclude this journey, remember that yoga is a powerful tool for empowering women's reproductive health. By integrating yoga into daily life, women can transform their physical, emotional, and spiritual wellbeing.

Key Takeaways

1. Yoga enhances reproductive health and hormone balance.

2. Mindfulness and self-awareness are crucial for women's wellbeing.

3. Yoga philosophy promotes self-love, acceptance, and empowerment.

4. Community support and resources foster long-term growth.

Empowering Women's Health Through Yoga

1. Breaks cycles of shame and stigma around reproductive health.

2. Fosters self-advocacy and informed decision-making.

3. Cultivates resilience and coping mechanisms.

4. Encourages holistic approach to health and wellness.

Conclusion

Yoga empowers women to take charge of their reproductive health, cultivating physical, emotional, and spiritual wellbeing. Remember, every breath, every pose, and every moment is an opportunity to transform and thrive.